The secret lies in mastering your BODY, turning it from a bicycle to a racecar, shack into a castle. You must first master the basics, which may take years. When you spend the entire day maintaining awareness while performing your daily tasks, you are ready to advance

HOW TO STAND

When relaxed, hands hang with palms facing the body

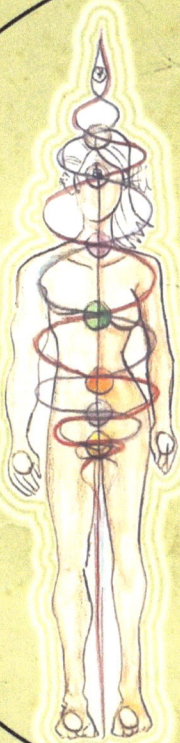

Shoulders pulled back slightly

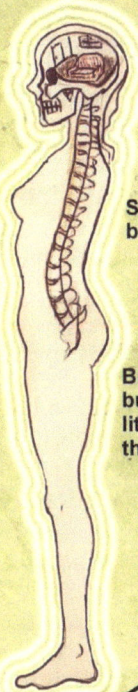

Bring belly button in just a little bit, keep it there all day.

Stand alert and ready for action, feet pointing straight ahead. Look down and check regularly

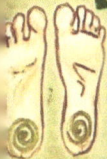

When energy is needed or feeling down, strike a heroic pose and feel the power and extra energy that comes with it!

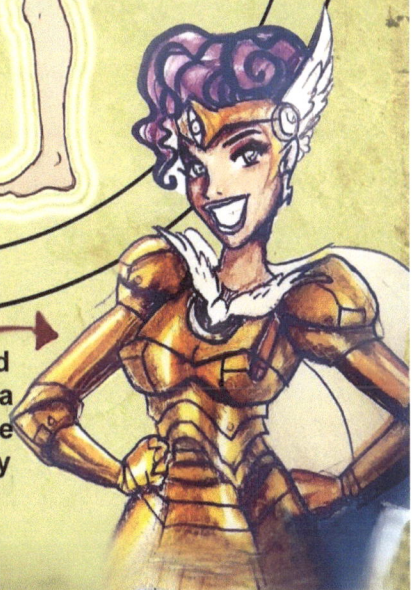

HOW TO STAND

Purpose

Keeping weight evenly displaced over both feet with hips, torso and head in optimal position promotes balance.

This will enable your human form to perform at super-human levels when ready.

WHAT TO EXPECT AFTER 1 YEAR:

Skills increase: Balance is also the key to finding proper rhythm when walking, running or performing ANY physical activity.

Rhythm leads to momentum and force production. Balance will allow you to control this force. This can be applied to strength, speed, acceleration, striking and endurance. and mental force...

Charisma / Confidence Increase:

It does not take an expert to see the difference in how a hero or authority figure stands and an average human. The hero stance is powerful for a reason, it works, it has an influence on the one who uses it and the ones who are witness to it. When those around you see this posture regularly you will be perceived differently. By friends as someone to admire and emulate... and by enemies and foes as someone to fear and not trifle with, especially the internal ones...

Luck Increase

It is not really luck, but to the average human it seems so. Balance brings awareness, internal and external. Chronic injuries do not exist, if they do the cause can be identified immediately and dealt with. Even thinking will quicken and headaches will diminish because of proper blood flow to the brain.

Proper balance will even help avoid accidents, causing the average human to believe luck is involved. Balance and awareness enables the hero to recognize and deal with unexpected obstacles. Especially the emotional ones.

STANDING

Directions: Throughout the day, whenever you find yourself standing, do a mental checklist of these 4 goals.

1. Head is up straight.

2. Bring the shoulders back and chest out.

3. Draw in the bellybutton just a little, keep it there as long as you can remember.

4. Look down randomly throughout the day to check that your feet are straight and your weight is even on both feet.

PURPOSE:

- Keeping weight evenly displaced over both feet with hips, torso and head in optimal position promotes balance.

- Keeping your feet pointed forward prevents problems in the knees, hips and lower back down the road. When your feet aren't straight, they must be turned on every step, which wastes milliseconds. Something a superhuman can't spare.

- Drawing in the belly button turns "on" the transverse abdominus muscle. This is your main core muscle which should always be "on" when you're active . Children all have it "on" but lose it from too much sitting.

- Head and spine always straight promotes nerve and blood flow to the head and prevents neck and shoulder deviations and pain.

Breathing at Rest

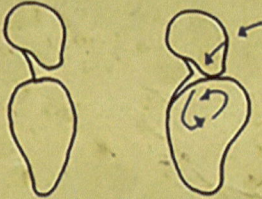

Most humans raise their chest when they breathe deep. This is the proper breathing for physical activity, keeping the belly in provides support for the core and lower back.

Conscious deep breathing

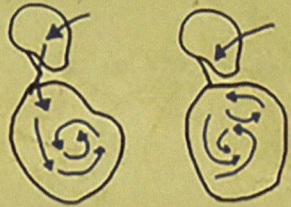

A SUPERHUMAN uses their belly like a balloon, which holds more air. They can also combine belly and chest inhale to get even more air.

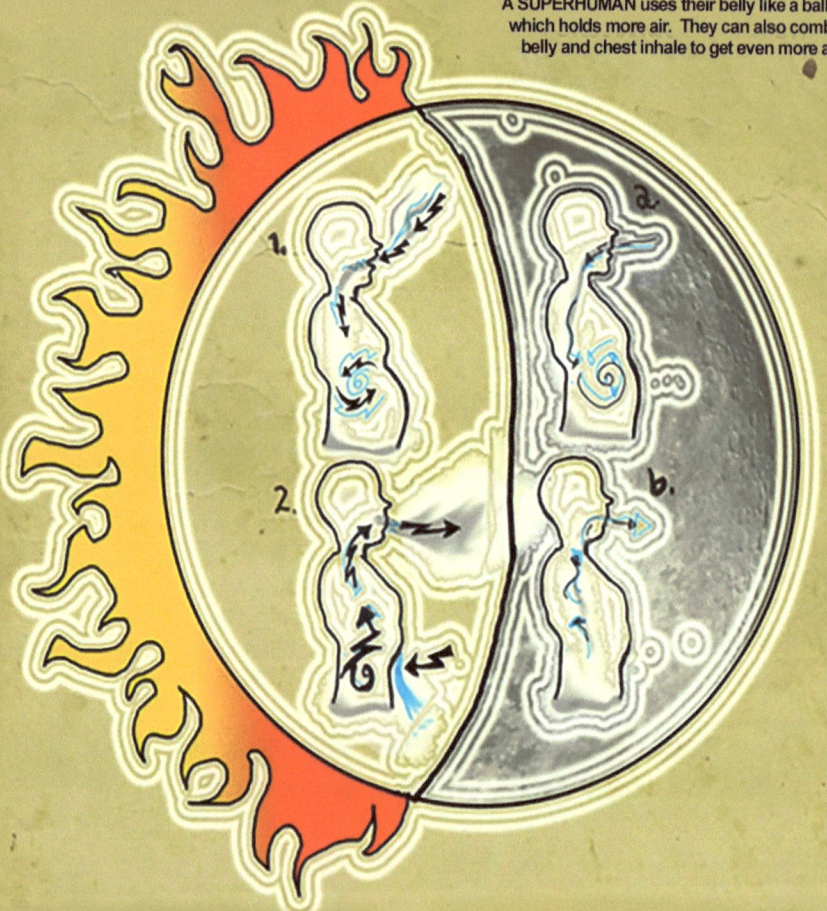

1. For energy during the day, inhale deep expanding the belly full of air.

2. Exhale quickly and forcefully bringing the belly button to the spine.
Do this just a few times at first

a. For relaxation, inhale deep through the nose.

b. Then let the air expel naturally with no effort like a balloon deflating. Be calm and aware of your breathing.

We all have 3 areas of the lung we can utilize for oxygen intake and most of us use only 2.

1. clavicular area around throat- for short shallow breathing like during intense exercise
2. chest area behind ribcage- where most of us breath at the moment. Seen in the rising and falling of chest.
3. diaphragm, abdominal- where the most air can be held. Seen as expansion and contraction of belly

It is not easy to change your breathing pattern after a lifetime doing it the wrong way, just take some time and imagine your belly is balloon that needs to be filled. Then fill it with air without raising the ribcage. The first exercise is be still and take 6 deep breaths focusing on ballooning abs on the inhale and exhaling by drawing abs in towards spine. Minimal effort should be used. This should be done whenever remembered.

Shallow breathing is associated with illness and disease. This is why a superhuman must control their breathing and posture before anything.

Alot of the body's functions are subject to cyclical rhythms and other outside influences out of our control. Breathing is the integral part of the mind-body interface. One that we can voluntarily control. To not use this interface to your advantage is neglectful and a misuse of the only body you have. If only one thing is taken from this book, it should be this section.

The body is at the mercy of cycles.

The cycles of the brains (thoughts) are connected to the cycles of the heart (emotion). Which are connected to the cycles of breathing.

Through aware breathing we gain access to aspects of our existence that normal humans don't have conscious control of!

It is like a cheat code for life and the first mandatory step for becoming superhuman.

HOW TO SIT

To be practiced every time you sit

When sitting a Superhuman does not flop down at the mercy of gravity.

1. Start from a standing position, draw in belly button, tighten core and slowly lower yourself to sitting.

2. Weight on heels the whole time. You should be able to stop and raise your toes any time on way down.

3. Your pelvic floor muscles are crucial, these are the muscles that are used when you have to use the toilet and hold it. As you lower yourself separate knees as you sit, stretching and tightening these muscles at the same time.

4. Keep your knees aligned with your feet.

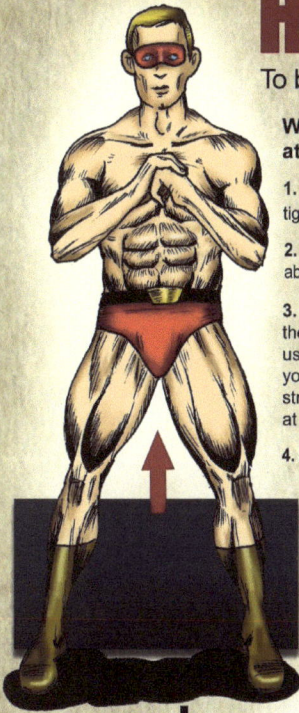

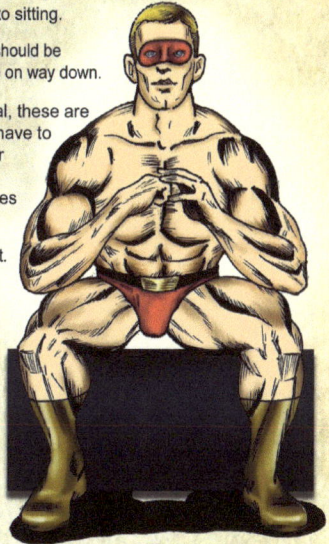

5. Keep shoulders between knees and hips until firmly down.

When arising do the same in reverse order.

Someone could kick a chair out from under a superhuman and they wouldn't spill a drop of their tea.

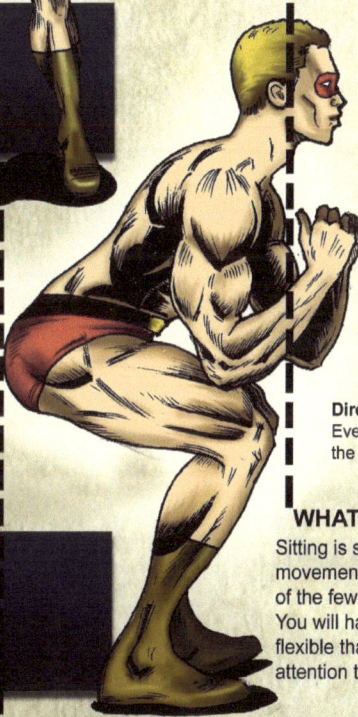

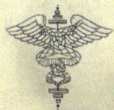

Directions:
Every time you sit remember and execute the 5 points above.

WHAT TO EXPECT AFTER A YEAR

Sitting is squatting, squatting is the foundation movement for humans. After a year you will be one of the few humans who do this movement properly. You will have less injuries, be stronger and more flexible than the average human, simply by paying attention to something you do everyday!

HOW TO WALK

To be practiced whenever you walk

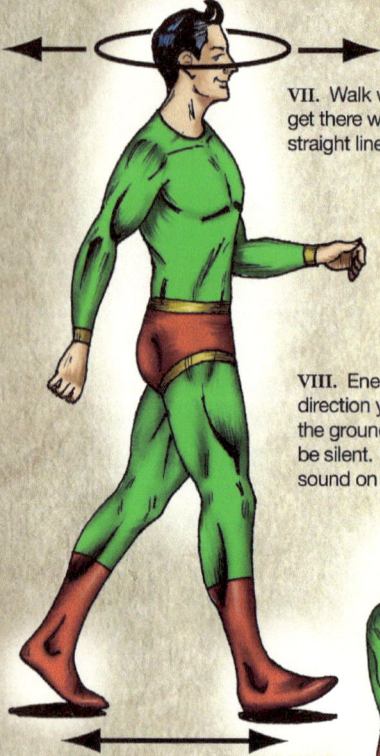

VII. Walk with purpose, know where you are going and get there with long smooth rhythmic strides. Follow a straight line to your destination.

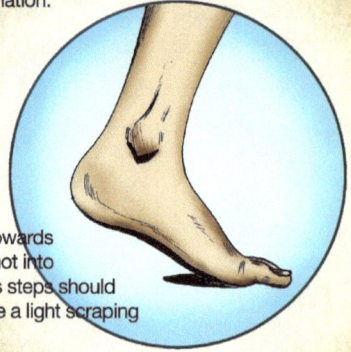

VIII. Energy directed towards direction you're going, not into the ground. This means steps should be silent. Except maybe a light scraping sound on end.

Keep head up. switch focus every few steps between: destination, ground in front of you and environment. A hero is never a victim of accidents or caught by surprise.

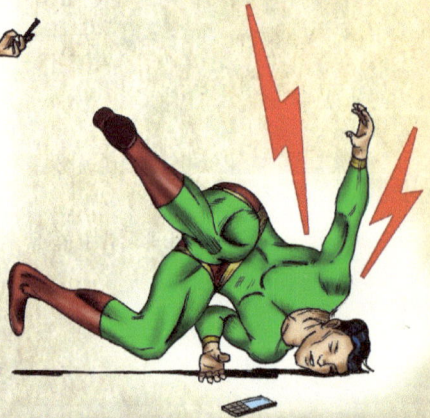

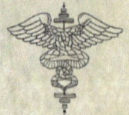

IX. Stride length is key to getting there and even rhythm will maximize speed and preserve energy.

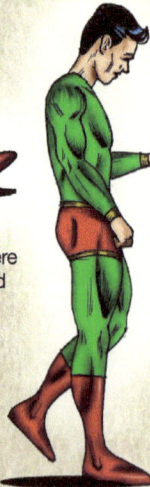

WALKING

Whenever walking, practice these 4 steps:

1. Practice walking with purpose. Rhythmic, long strides will teach the mind focus and the body proper mechanics for moving and running. Those who see this take notice, giving you a psychological advantage over regular humans. Combine with a heroic posture for best effect. . This teaches how to manipulate energy and use it to complete certain goals.

2. Keeping your head up and paying attention to the path ahead is the beginning of super sense training. Where you will be able to identify dangerous situations and environmental hazards before an average human would. Like a seasoned policeman, soldier, fighter or spy.

3: Reducing sound when walking or running reduces ground impact. Too much impact adds up over millions of steps over a lifetime. Reducing impact when walking and running prevents wear on joints and prevents injuries through life.

4. Focusing on stride length keeps you strong, flexible and efficient.

HOW TO RUN

1. Elbows always bent to save time and energy each stride. Lean forward when starting to reach maximum speed faster.

2. Lift Toe as soon as foot leaves ground, throwing opposite elbow up and toward center of chest, hand should be open relaxed and at midline at top.

3. Just like walking, stay in straight line to destination, focusing on stride length and rhythm. The quieter your steps, the more efficient your running. Stride length is the key to getting there

Directions:
After thorough warm up practice running on
leg (foundation) day.5-10 sprints between 20 and 100 meters.
Start at 60% of max speed and add intensity every week
until you are able to run 100% effort without injury.
Increase distance over time. take One to three months off
of 100% running every year, once consistent.

HOW TO RUN

To be practiced on leg day or whenever running

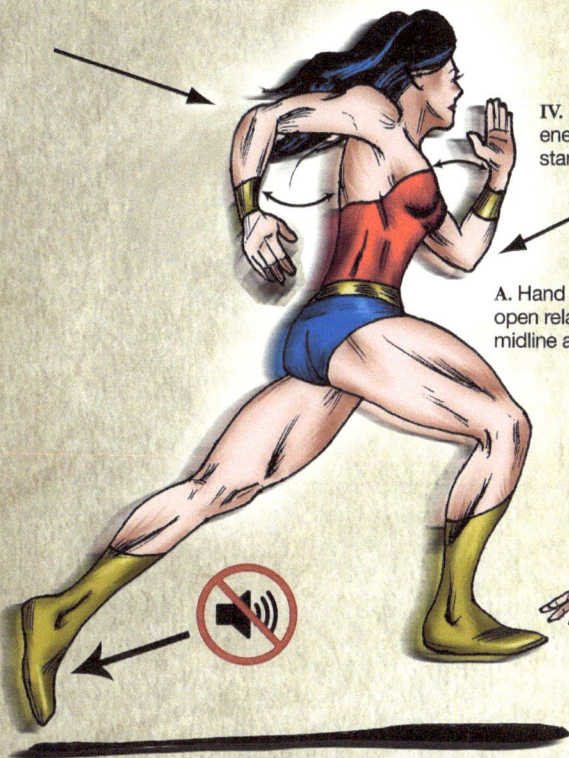

IV. Elbows always bent to save time and energy each stride. Lean forward when starting to reach maximum speed faster.

A. Hand should be open relaxed and at midline at top.

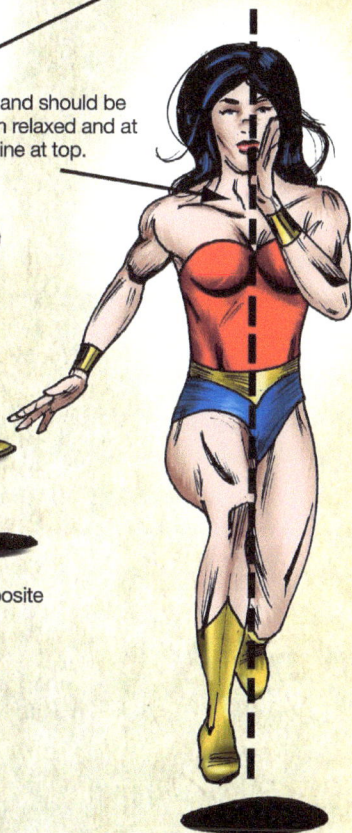

V. Lift toe as soon as foot leaves ground, throwing opposite elbow up and toward center of chest.

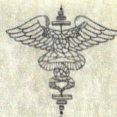

Cold Showers

If you can not start right away, just finish
a hot shower with a cold rinse. Add
more time in cold every time until you
are used to it.

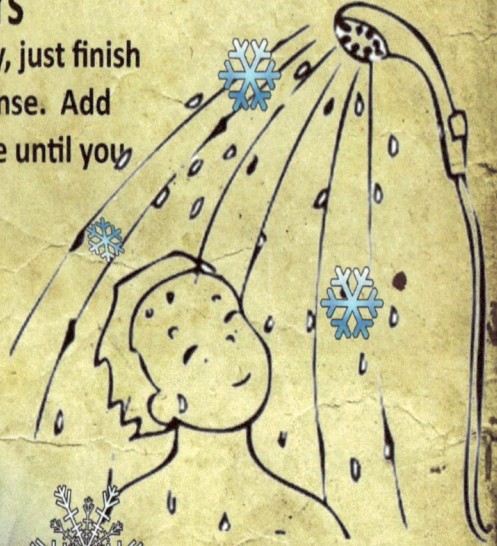

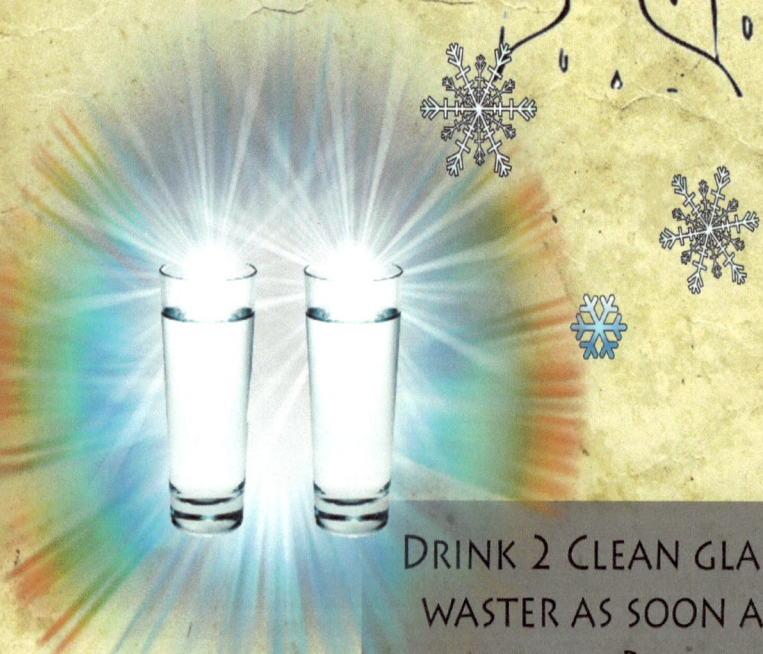

DRINK 2 CLEAN GLASSES OF
WASTER AS SOON AS YOU
WAKE UP, BEFORE ANY-
THING ELSE IS DONE.

Go barefoot as often as you can.

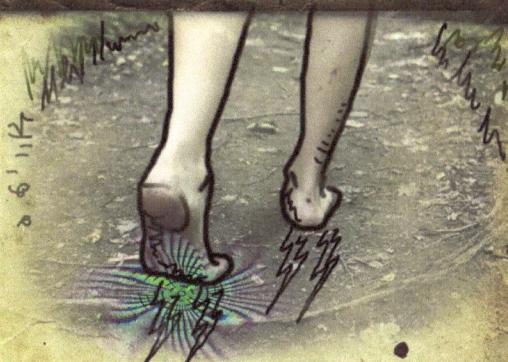

Muscles in the feet need to be trained also. Enables you to absorb energy of the Earth. Anyone can feel it, just take your shoes off and walk on earth or grass. That good feeling is earth energy flowing into you. This is why water and wind feel good also.

Wake up when sun comes up.

Expose skin to sun during day

Go to sleep when sun goes down or soon after. Stay away from too much light at night.

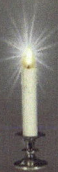

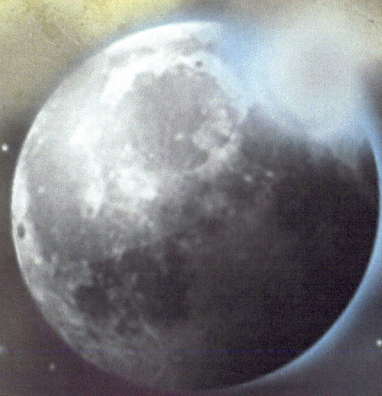

HOW TO ADD MUSCLE

DAMAGE RECOVER ADAPT

The following pages are top secret Superhero Training Manual techniques to add muscle and strength for beginners. You will need 5 minutes, 2-3 times a week to achieve a strength and muscularity level in one year that you did not think possible.

You will be among the 1% strongest humans in your age group pound for pound by years end.

First you must identify the main goal, adding strength and muscle! It seems logical, but everyone is more concerned about the workout, falsely assuming more is better. They are wrong.

Second you must break down how it is done. Here it is:

1. Impose a stress on the muscle that causes DAMAGE to the nerves, muscle tissue and stresses the bones other bodily systems. (workout)

2. Rest and let muscles, nerves, bones and other bodily systems heal. RECOVERY

3. After recovery allow body extra day or two to ADAPT this is adding muscle, nerve connections, blood vessels and bone material to make sure same workout is easier next time.

Remember, the workout is DAMAGING tissue, so doing any workout DAMAGE before RECOVERY or ADAPTATION is wrong.
It is the same as getting a sun-tan.

PUSHING STRENGTH

You don't need dozens of movements to develop strength and size. In the pushing series, we use simple horizontal and vertical movements work the pushing muscles.

1. **Chest** (Pushing horizontal from torso)

2. **Shoulders** (Pushing overhead)

3. **Triceps** (Straightening arm at elbow)

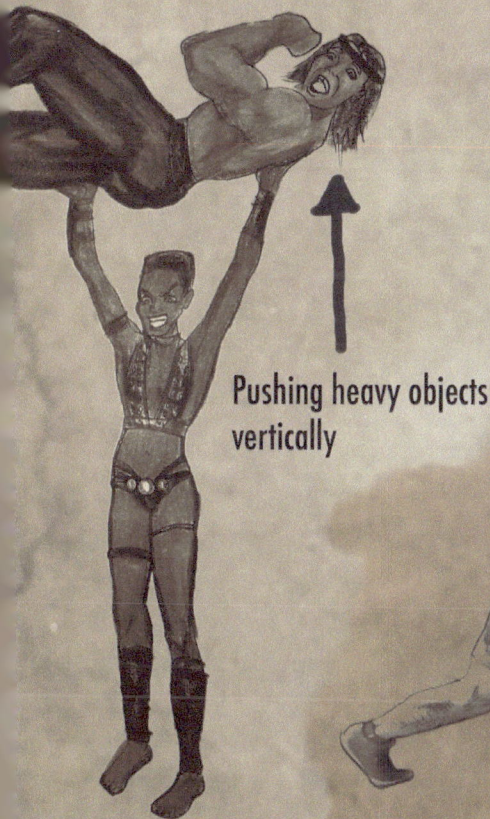

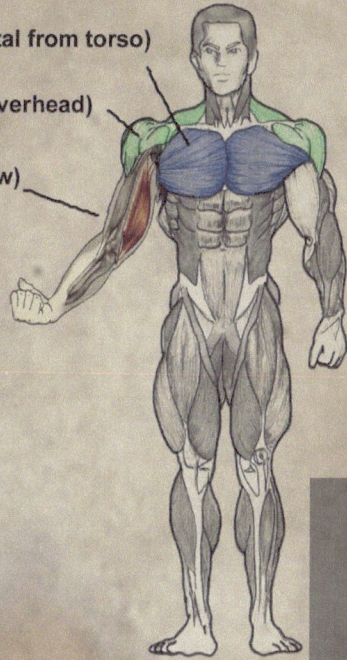

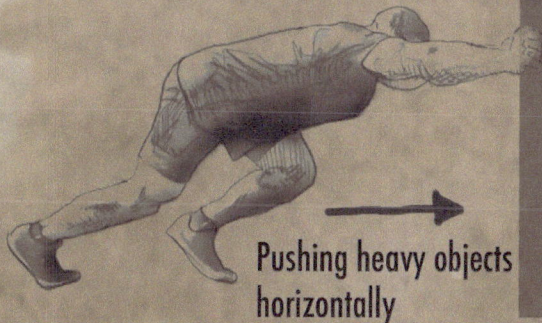

Pushing heavy objects vertically

Pushing heavy objects horizontally

PUSHING DAY WORKOUT

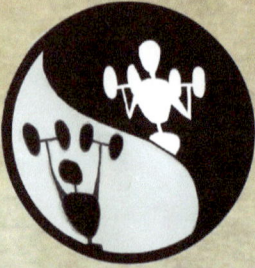

- Pushups, dips, handstands, bands cables and machines all work.
- To maximize the workouts obey they following procedures for body alignment and rep range.

Remember, after warm-up, **only 1 set of as many repetitions as possible per exercise**

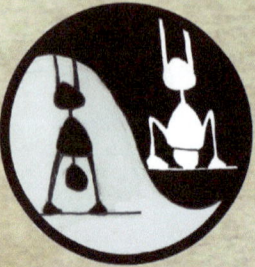

1. Retract scapula- bring shoulder blades together; following this action the chest will rise.

2. A good cue is to think chest high shoulders back. This is the proper form, there is a tendency to round the shoulders near exhaustion so pay attention to this.

3. Keep chest high- Related to the scapular retraction, it puts the pushing muscles in position for maximum contraction and the shoulders in the right position to avoid excess stress.

4. Keep abs and core tight by drawing them in. Start by the exhaling all air and drawing bellybutton to spine, just as you do with breathing for energy. Hold the belly in the drawn in position as you perform your exercises.

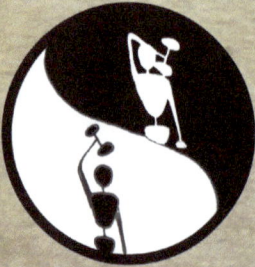

5. Find optimum range. There is a certain point in any exercise range of motion, where it becomes inefficient and dangerous. Your range will be the range that's easiest for you. This is your strongest range, it can increase as weeks go by. You may start pushups only going a quarter of the way down at first. Later you can work on range and repetitions.

6. Knowing how to establish a mind muscle connection is crucial. When pushing horizontally-àuse chest muscles (pecs) when pushing overhead use shoulder muscles and bring in bellybutton to support spine. If you feel it more in the arms you may have to adjust your form.

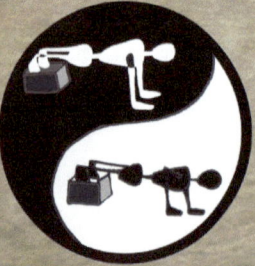

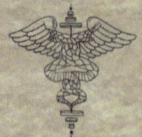

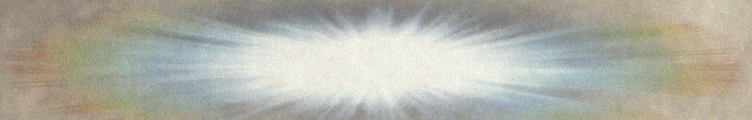

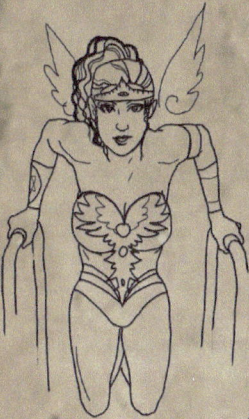

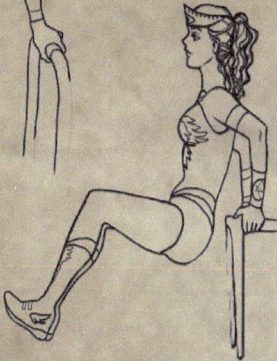

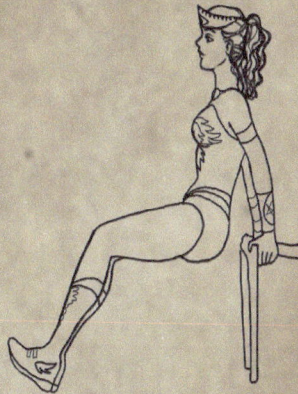

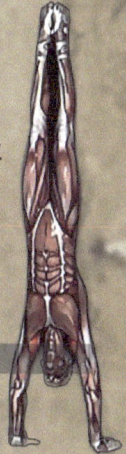

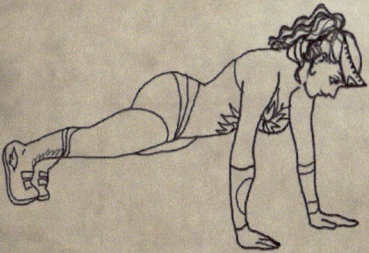

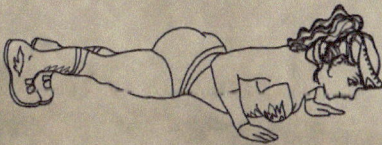

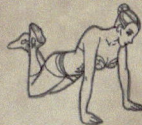

It's OK to use your knees!

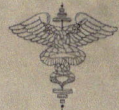

PRESSES

CHEST PRESSES - Incline, decline, flat, dumbells and barbells are the base of a solid chest workout. Beginners can also use pushups, bands cables and machines and still get results. To maximize the workouts obey they following procedures for body alignment and rep range.

1. Retract scapula - Bring the shoulder blades together, following this action will make the chest rise. A good cue is to think -chest high, shoulders back. This is the proper form. There is a tendency to round the shoulders near exhaustion so pay attention to this.

2. Keep the chest high - Related to the scapular retraction, it puts the pectorals in position for maximum contraction and the shoulders in the right position to avoid excess stress.

3. Keep abs and core tight by drawing them in.

(The above guidelines go for every upper body exercise. It puts the spine in an ideal position to generate force and prevent injury.)

4. Find the optimum range - There is a certain point when lowering the weight on a chest press, where the pectorals lose leverage and the resistance accelerates down. This is clearly visible when you see bench pressers repping to the chest. Stop the repetition just above this point to maintain tension on the pectorals.

5. Keep your wrists straight. In beginners, you might see the wrist break. The palms end up facing up and the stress is shifted to the wrist instead of lining up with the forearm.

6. The starting position for a press is somewhere between just below the lower pec and the neck. The strongest position is somewhere in between.

Knowing how to establish a mind-muscle connection is crucial. Compare the feeling of the pecs between a regular bench press and a dumbell press using the techniques above. It should be immediately apparent. The techniques above will produce better results. Look for and feel the "pump".

Pulling Day

Pulling strength is another simple way to build strength and size. Find fun ways to use your pulling muscles like climbing a tree!

1. **Latisimuss** dorsi (wings),

2. **Back** muscles

3. Forearms and Grip.

4. Biceps,

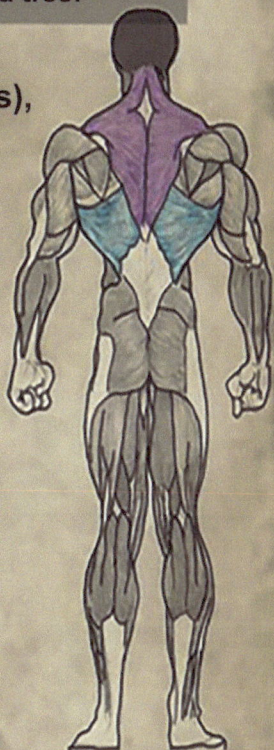

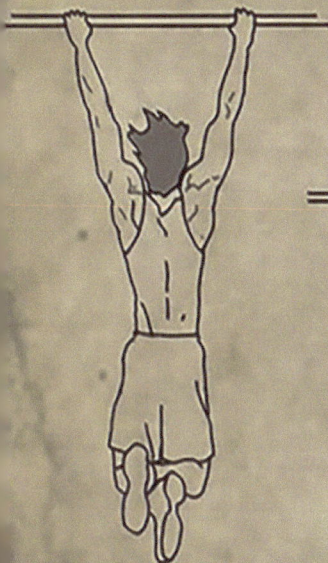

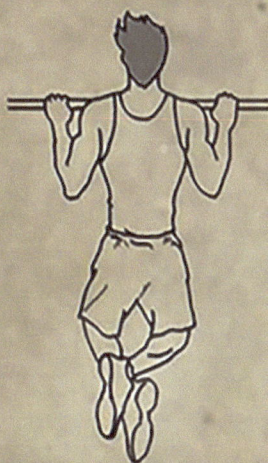

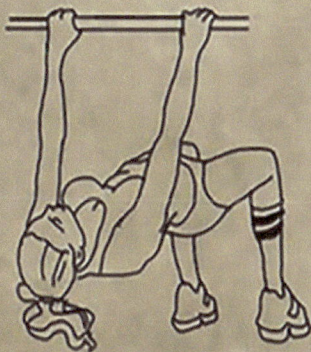

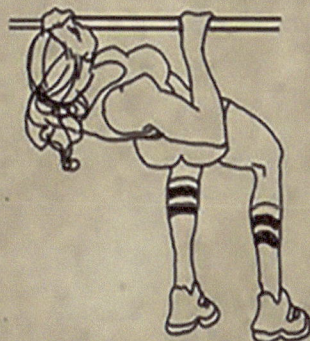

PULLING

The pulling group is the largest muscle group of the body, responsible for posture and is the base for all shoulder movements.

The horizontal pull towards the body improves posture. Make sure to squeeze shoulder blades together and focus on bringing elbows back and chest up.

PULLING DAY

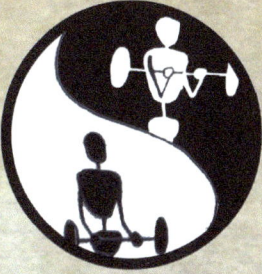

1. The pulling group is the largest muscle group of the body, responsible for posture and is the base for all shoulder movements, grip, hand strength and the most famous muscle of all, biceps. Treat it as such.

2. The horizontal pull toward body improves posture, if you make sure to squeeze shoulder blades together and focus on bringing elbows back and chest up.

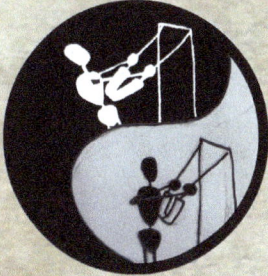

3. The vertical pull builds the latisimuss dorsi, the biggest muscle of the upper body. Can be done at any playground. If you cannot do a pull-up, hang, if you cannot hang, hold bar and pull hard as you can with feet on ground.

4. Grip and hand position are important. Beginners should use parallel or underhand grip. Overhand grip is hardest and should be used later. A good practice is to do one of each overhand first.

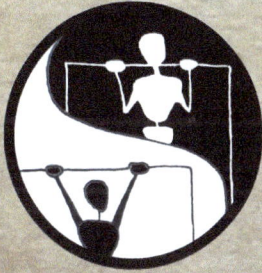

5. The mind muscle connection is crucial, focus on pulling with upper arms and elbows and squeezing shoulder blades down and back. The goal is to feel it in the back muscles and not the arms.

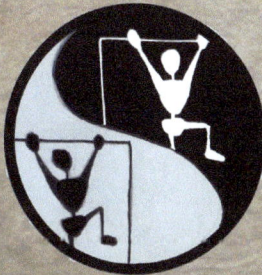

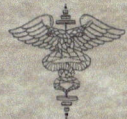

CALENDAR
Time to go to work

The following portion of this manual is the the most important.
This is where you put what you have learned into action.
It is very simple, commit to practice one or all of the following.

Standing: At least once during day look down and make sure feet are pointed straight ahead, belly button drawn in, shoulders back and head straight (4 cues)

Breathing: at least once per day practice inhaling and have belly expand and exhale by drawing abdomen in strongly 7 x.

Sitting: At least once per day, when you sit make sure you tighten pelvic floor muscles and core and align knees with toes as you sit and get up in the same way.

Walking: Once during day, while walking, focus on gliding, long strides, posture and silent steps

Sleeping/ avoiding artificial light: If you go to sleep not too long after dark and wake up to get morning sun.

2 glasses of water immediately after waking

cold thermogenisis: cold rinse or shower or not using heater or heavy coat to stay warm as winter approaches

walk, sit or stand barefoot on earth, grass or even cement for an hour

If you perform the tasks described below during the day put a red "x" on your calendar. It could be one behavior, but if it is more than one, all must be completed before bed to earn that red "x".
To become Superhuman, you must put together long strings of "x'"s on your calendar. If you miss a day, pick up again the next day.

Those that can fill 11 months of unbroken chain of "x's will receive Volume 2 free.
Send email to **LankfordICSP@gmail.com** and prepare for advanced training!

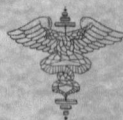

Month/Year:

Sunday	Monday	Tuesday	Wednesday	Thursday	Friday	Saturday

The Musical Mind (http://people.upei.ca/ajncli)

First Month Challenge!
Send me your results on social media!

Month/Year:

Sunday	Monday	Tuesday	Wednesday	Thursday	Friday	Saturday

The Musical Mind (http://people.upei.ca/izjnck)

Second Month Challenge!
Are you seeing any progress?

Month/Year:

Sunday	Monday	Tuesday	Wednesday	Thursday	Friday	Saturday

3rd Month Challenge!
90 days and you should be feeling like a new you!
Make sure to take pictures.

Month/Year:

Sunday	Monday	Tuesday	Wednesday	Thursday	Friday	Saturday

The Musical Mind (http://people.upei.ca/znel)

Fourth Month Challenge!
Have you made consistant habits and changes?

Month/Year:

Sunday	Monday	Tuesday	Wednesday	Thursday	Friday	Saturday

The Musical Mind (http://people.upei.ca/szjneli)

5th Month Challenge!
You are almost halfway!

Month/Year:

Sunday	Monday	Tuesday	Wednesday	Thursday	Friday	Saturday

6th Month Challenge!
You have officially made it to the halfway mark.
Lets see some transformation photos!

Month/Year:

Sunday	Monday	Tuesday	Wednesday	Thursday	Friday	Saturday

The Musical Mind (http://people.upei.ca/zajacb/)

Seventh Month Challenge!
Keep going to full on Superhuman status!

Month/Year:

Sunday	Monday	Tuesday	Wednesday	Thursday	Friday	Saturday

8th Month Challenge!

Need help? Find other superhumans on our facebook page and get support to continue your transformation

Month/Year:

Sunday	Monday	Tuesday	Wednesday	Thursday	Friday	Saturday

Ninth Month Challenge!
A new baby superhuman is born!

Month/Year:

Sunday	Monday	Tuesday	Wednesday	Thursday	Friday	Saturday

10th Month Challenge!
Share your story with others now!

Month/Year:

Sunday	Monday	Tuesday	Wednesday	Thursday	Friday	Saturday

11th Month Challenge!
Home-stretch, by now you have officially integrated the lifestyle of a superhuman.